winner
michigan writers cooperative press
2025 creative nonfiction contest

Gifts from the Edge of Life
Reflections of a grateful nurse
Wendy Gilbert Gronbeck

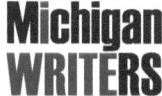

Copyright © 2025 by Wendy Gilbert Gronbeck. All rights reserved.

Michigan Writers Cooperative Press
P. O. Box 2355
Traverse City, Michigan 49685

ISBN-13: 978-1-950744-24-4

Book design by Amy Hansen

Contents

Foreword	1
Hazel: Teachable Moments	2
Lorena: The View from Here	6
Paulette: Trooper	8
Barbara: Stylin'	10
Marne: Those !&?@#!#%& Nurses!	13
Margie: Watch Your Step	16
Jenni: On Second Thought	19
Daniel: The Finale	22
Edna: Cold Comfort	24
David: Facing the Music	28
Annie: A Father's Gift	30
Ida: Hide the Kids!	32
Margaret: The Special Gift	34
Acknowledgements	37
About the Creative Nonfiction Judge	38
About the Author	39
About Michigan Writers Cooperative Press	40
Other Titles Available	41

GIFTS FROM THE EDGE OF LIFE
Reflections of a grateful nurse

Foreword

The drippy, smelly, gorier aspects of nursing are not for everyone, and working with patients facing terminal illnesses may be even less appealing. Yet every day, oncology and hospice nurses stand right there at the edge of life, face-to-face with mortality. Some difficult stuff happens out there. Your shoes get sticky, and your heart gets broken. Maybe that's why sooner or later, most nurses are asked, "How can you stand to be a nurse?" It's a darn good question. The answer is: sometimes, right in the midst of ducking airborne bodily fluids and arguing with penny-pinching administrators, something special happens, a rare moment when the life of a vulnerable patient and the life of a nurse intersect. When that happens, we are privy to precious moments that teach, touch, and inspire. That's why we can stand to be nurses. My life was profoundly changed by people I cared for on an inpatient oncology unit and in homes and care centers as a hospice nurse. Some were gems and some were corkers, and I remember them fondly in the following stories.

Identifying details have been well muddled to protect identities. Key events, quotations, and impact on this nurse have not.

Hazel: Teachable Moments

When I was a child, my mother told me to stay at the table until I ate at least one bite of liver. I told her I'd rather grow up at the kitchen table than eat liver. This early-onset contrariness may explain my affinity for the more cantankerous patients, those who railed against the injustice, fear, and the indignities of illness, treatments, and dying. I loved to care for those "go out swinging" folks. One was Hazel.

Eighty-year-old Hazel was referred to hospice even though she still was able to fix simple meals and putter around her yard. She agreed to accept help managing medications and washing her hair, but nothing more.

On my first visit, I opened the door to a small woman in a stained sweatsuit. Her face was peppered with dark spots, some of which I suspected were skin cancers, but that was the least of her problems – she had advanced colon cancer. Hazel's gray hair was short, most likely a do-it-yourself haircut. She motioned for me to come in, and I took one step forward and two steps back. Hazel lived with multiple cats and no litter boxes, but they found the overstuffed chairs in the living room to be a good substitute. Trash bags lined the dining room, and clothes were piled on the bed. I don't mind clutter – the trunk of my car was jammed with bandages and urinals, IV poles and blue bed pads. I knew the skinny legs of a commode sticking up through the moon roof didn't look at all professional. So, Hazel's clutter was bearable, but the caustic, feline fragrance was a surprise, even for a nurse's nose. Grateful it was summer, I suggested we chat on the front porch with its morning sunlight and the scent of roses climbing a nearby trellis.

The first few visits to Hazel proved a challenge. She was suspicious of all these strangers asking personal questions. The parade of nurses, social workers, and chaplains interrupted her private life, and she wasn't sure what we were up to. Did we want to put her in a nursing home? Make her get rid of the cats? If we asked a personal question, she'd snap "What's that matter to you?" Hazel was dead set against having a nurse's aide give her a bath, so I made a deal: if she tried it one time and didn't like it, I'd stop bugging her. That trial technique almost always works. Hazel enjoyed the soothing baths and the lotion massaged into her clean skin. By moving slowly and giving her options, we gained her trust.

During the summer, I watched Hazel relinquish one chunk of independence and privacy after another, and my heart ached for her. The challenge was balancing Hazel's right to choose how she lived with my professional responsibility for her safety and health. I imagined someone inspecting my house, pointing out that murderous throw rug in the hall or cheese that is not just aged, but should be pronounced dead. I would be boarding up my doors.

Shortly after Hazel was admitted to hospice, we were contacted by a physician who was teaching first-year medical students about end-of-life care. She asked if her students could chat with one of our patients. I consulted with Hazel, and she agreed. Personally, I couldn't wait to see how the students responded to Hazel's environment. They'd been in a sterile hospital setting, and this was their first adventure in home care.

Hazel watched the professor and five students in short white coats parade up the walk. She opened the door and offered her guests a chair. Their smiles froze. We had not yet tackled Hazel's cat problem, and only a seriously insensate person would sink into one of those stained, frothy chairs. The students murmured a few "Oh, we're okays" and leaned against the walls. Hazel took around a plate of cookies. There was no getting out of this. I saw several cookies slip into lab coat pockets.

These students were not just inexperienced as physicians; they were inexperienced as human beings. One was peering at an old upright piano, perhaps confused because the keys were so dusty you couldn't tell the black keys from the white ones. Another stared at the row of flowerpots on the windowsill, each with one brown, dried-up stem.

Hazel, meanwhile, was excited to have an audience and chatted enthusiastically about how long she'd lived in the house and how much she knew about the neighborhood's history. She was on a roll when the professor interrupted her, because these students needed to learn about dying, not living. She dug right in.

"Tell us what it's like to find out you're dying, Hazel." As an aside, she turned to her students and whispered, "*This is a teachable moment.*" I cringed. If someone pressured me to conduct my own wake in front of strangers, I would have shown her to the door. Hazel simply gave her a puzzled look and went right on talking about her parents settling in this city and changes she'd seen in her lifetime. Every time she got going, the physician would redirect her to her terminal state.

"Do you think about it much?"

"Are you depressed?"

"Is it scary to be dying?" Part of me wanted Hazel to say, "Hell, no. Dying is a blast! Whyever do you ask?"

Periodically, the physician pointed out those "teachable moments" as though Hazel wasn't right there in the room with us. Hazel straightened herself up, sitting taller, as though summoning strength to ignore the physician. She continued with stories about her life, despite attempts to focus on her death. She was trying to show she mattered, that she was a person with a history and a place in the community. The professor attempted one last time to lead her to death's door, and Hazel bestowed upon her a teachable moment of her own.

"Hey, I know I'm gonna die," she said. "Until then, I'd just as soon not be thinking about it all the time."

Hazel, like many in her age group, was firm in her resolve to remain in her home. There are risk factors professionals use to assess the likelihood a person will or won't be able to remain home successfully. Hazel ticked off all the negative indicators and a few more, but those list makers had not met the likes of her. I don't think she was related to the Wallendas, but she stumbled and fell around her house much like the unfortunate aerial troop, rebounding off door jambs and furniture, occasionally tripping over a cat. One day, she called and told me she'd fallen and cut her forehead.

Hazel greeted me at the door with a red slit above her eyebrow. Although it wasn't bleeding much, it did need stitches. She was wearing her pink nightie and one earring, and she jolly well wasn't about to go to the ER until she found the other one. You could throw an earring into the crowd at the Super Bowl and have a better chance of retrieving it than you would in Hazel's bedroom. I sorted through bedding and fearlessly dropped to my knees to check under the bed. After half an hour, I told her we needed to get her head repaired.

I sat on the edge of the bed to help Hazel get dressed. She took off her nightie, and when she turned her bare back to me, there it was! One gold earring. The sharp earring post was pressed well into her bottom. I told Hazel she was a long way from starring in The Princess and the Pea. I retrieved the earring, she put it on, and off we went. Yes, it did go right from her bum to her ear lobe.

In the ER, a young doc examined Hazel and stitched her up, then he closed the chart and spoke in his most sincere doctor voice.

"Hazel, I see you've fallen more than a few times. Maybe it's time we think about a nursing home."

Hazel sat up and leaned in, her nose inches from his.

"Young man," she said, "there's worse things than stitches."

Lorena: The View from Here

Anyone who thinks the first year of marriage is difficult ought to consider Lorena and Dan's first few months as newlyweds. Shortly after their wedding, Lorena was diagnosed with a cancer that was curable, but the treatment would make it impossible for her to become pregnant. This was bitter news for twenty-somethings anxious to start a family. I got to know this lovely couple during her surgery and several rounds of chemotherapy. Lorena was open about her sadness at never carrying a baby, but I saw no self-pity, no *"Why me?"* She and her husband focused on getting through the treatments.

One morning as I walked down the hall, I saw Dan sitting at his wife's bedside. She smiled and looked past him at the sky outside her window. At her age, I would have been curled up in a ball on my bed, cloaked in grief for the babies I yearned for so powerfully. It's possible I could not have weathered such a storm, certainly not with the calm these two were showing. Yes, Lorena's brown eyes were sad, but they also had a peaceful expression. Her husband brushed her oak-brown hair, taking his time, running his hand over each lock as he smoothed it. Here was a man showing his wife *I am with you, and we will be okay.*

After chemotherapy was complete, we didn't see Lorena and Dan again. This is good news, because it means the patient came to the outpatient clinic for a check-up, and her medical team found no need for further treatment.

About ten years after Lorena's stay on our unit, I was at a concert in a large performing arts center. As I settled in my seat, someone tapped me on the shoulder. I turned and looked into those kind, brown eyes from several years ago. Her hair was in the same style – she hadn't aged much, but it was that palpable connection with the man standing next to her that I recognized.

"You probably don't remember us," she said.

Nurses generally see patients in bed in a drab hospital room, wearing hospital gowns, hair askew or missing. They're sleeping or throwing up, so when we run into them years later in Target, we may not recognize them right away. Sometimes our memories fail us, and it's embarrassing: *I inserted a catheter into you, but I can't remember your face.*

Now, we were in a concert hall with gold-trimmed columns and a red velvet curtain, and they were a handsome couple in evening attire. I was grateful that even in this setting, her name popped right into my head.

"Lorena! How are you?" I was thrilled to see her healthy and happy at a concert. She told me she and Dan had adopted a ten-year-old girl and then discovered she had a genetic disorder that would cause her body and mind to deteriorate over the next few years. The child would require constant care, perhaps indefinitely.

My stomach clenched. How unfair is a universe that takes away this woman's ability to carry a child and then punishes her generous spirit with a situation like this? Lorena proceeded to tell me how unfair it was. I was about to be schooled on perspective as something one chooses.

"*This* is why I was spared," she said. "I was meant to care for this child. Imagine her life if she'd remained in an institution." *Imagine*, indeed! Imagine how my view of the world expanded because of Lorena. That very morning, I'd yelled at my perfectly healthy son for sniffing through the laundry basket looking for his least dirty soccer shirt, not exactly a crisis compared to Lorena's situation.

I don't know if I heard the New York Philharmonic or Sweet Honey in the Rock at that concert, but I will never forget the love and humanity of the young couple seated across the aisle.

Paulette: Trooper

Paulette came to our unit looking, as my mother-in-law used to say, kinda tough. Her hair was dirty as were her clothes, and pain gripped her face, making her appear older than her thirty years. As we walked down the hall, I asked her if she had any children. She said she had two girls, six and seven, but it was clear she wasn't interested in chit-chat. When we came to her room, she disappeared into the clean bedding and curled up, knees to chin.

Paulette's advanced fallopian tube cancer was raging, and she was in serious trouble. I asked if her girls were with their dad during her hospital stay, and she peered out the window and said, "I don't even know their dads' last names." She was a single mom, she said, and traveled with a circus, managing make-up and costumes for the performers, barely supporting her family. She said the circus people were watching her children for her. Paulette had no healthcare benefits, no time off, no chance to make appointments for regular check-ups. Her life consisted of moving on and getting by. The word *circus* conjured up pictures of bearded ladies and men on stilts chasing bears in tutus, not a great place to raise children. My biases steamed through me like a hot flash, but soon I saw Paulette as the desperate young mother she was.

The immediate problem for Paulette was out-of-control pain. I had seen her scans. Cancer had infiltrated much of her pelvic cavity, and she was suffering every kind of pain – bone, nerve, and visceral, and it was constant. Being in the room with her as she cried, writhed, and occasionally screamed was unbearable. I knew her cries would upset patients in nearby rooms, making them wonder if this would happen to them, so I closed the door.

We increased the dose of Paulette's pain meds, but after several days, hadn't made enough progress. I took her pain home with me at night and thought about it first thing in the morning.

Before Paulette came to us, I had completed an evening course called Hypnosis for Symptom Relief. I knew no one could hypnotize me – that is, I thought I knew. In fact, at our first class, I went under like a rock in the river. When the instructor told me something was pushing my hand up in the air, I raised it like an excited third grader who finally knows the answer. Despite my negligible experience in that class, I thought I might give hypnosis a try with Paulette, since nothing else was working. Hypnosis is like deep meditation, and I doubted she could settle enough to listen, but she said she'd try anything.

I talked Paulette through some images, and she went into a deeply relaxed state. Her respirations slowed, and the cries and moans stopped. I was thrilled. I sat by her bed, grateful for this moment of peace, quite pleased with myself.

About twenty minutes later, all hell broke loose. Paulette sat bolt upright and started screaming loudly. I feared she was having a psychotic break, and I had caused it. Who did I think I was, playing with fire, not knowing what I was doing? I was about to call the psych nurses for help when Paulette quit yelling and just sat there, smiling and calm.

"Sorry to yell," she said. "That's the first time I've been without pain in months."

My heart rate didn't settle down for the rest of the shift. I should never have tried a new skill on someone so vulnerable.

I watched Paulette head for the elevator with her discharge instructions in hand, quite sure the remainder of her young life would be dreadful. We provided pain medications and referrals for various social services, but Paulette likely would not or could not access any of those resources. What would become of her children? Should I have called Child Protective Services? Why didn't we involve the hospital social workers more?

There are so many ways to feel inadequate when dealing with life's extreme situations day after day. This internal wrestling match between feeling like you should have done more and accepting one's limitations is exhausting.

I threw Paulette's chart into the discharge basket. Now, she was just a medical record, but somewhere, thirty years before, another nurse had welcomed a beautiful, newborn baby girl. She would be called Paulette.

Barbara: Stylin'

Barbara was a farmer, a big, strong woman with ruddy cheeks and a knee-slappin' sense of humor. Before her first chemotherapy treatment, she and I were reviewing side-effects and came to the dreaded hair-loss section. Most women find it devastating to lose their hair, because it pastes a big "cancer patient" label on you, one for everyone to see or pretend not to see. Barbara didn't seem concerned, but I wondered if her nonchalance would falter when she saw those first few locks come off on her comb.

When Barbara did lose her hair that first time, she remained unconcerned. She just wanted to put on her "I Am the Farmer's Daughter" hat and get back on her tractor. Over the next few years, she had periods of remission, then recurrence, another round of chemo, and each time, the hair loss. It never rattled her. "It'll grow back," she said. "I'll sprinkle a little fertilizer on my head."

For three years Barbara was in remission. Then, her name appeared on our admission list once again. I loved seeing her but wished this spirited woman could just live her country life in peace. She reported to the desk and said, "Here we go again." This time she was wearing an "I Like to Play in the Dirt" cap. When she removed it, everyone in the nursing station froze. Pens stopped writing, charts hovered aloft, the phone slipped from the clerk's ear. Three years was more than enough time to regrow a full head of hair, but that wasn't at all what we were looking at. Instead, jagged tufts of hair dotted Barbara's scalp here and there. She was Chia Barbara, and this was *before* chemo.

Barbara laughed at our mass paralysis and fluffed up a few

tufts like a movie star tossing her hair for the camera. When she'd told her grandchildren she needed more chemo and would lose her hair again, they'd asked if they could give her a haircut. She said, "Why not? Gonna lose it anyway." So, with their dull, plastic scissors, they crafted this dome of periodic stubble on their grandma's head.

We all laughed with Barbara. That is, everyone except one resident sitting at the back of the nursing station. She was the color of the white wall behind her.

"Barbara," she said, "I don't know how to tell you this. You're getting a new chemo drug, and it *doesn't* make your hair fall out."

We all swung back around to see how this was going to land. Barbara slapped the counter and laughed until she snorted. I guess wrangling 600 lb. hogs makes you tough.

I don't know if Barbara enjoyed a long life on her beloved farm. I do know that in her lifetime, she harvested far more than soybeans and corn. The way she faced challenges isn't innate – it was a decision. When self-pity or pettiness infect my attitude, the memory of Barbara's spirit is the perfect antidote.

Marne: Those !&?@#!#%& Nurses!

Marne was studying to become an agronomist and had just begun her junior year in college. She had big plans for organizing farm women into a powerful lobby, but now she faced a much bigger challenge. She arrived on our unit in a state of panic over newly diagnosed cervical cancer. It was caught early and was very curable, but after hearing, "You have cancer," nearly everyone is gripped by fear. Marne was a twenty-year-old facing a life-threatening situation, so no wonder she was terrified.

The plan for Marne was Cesium implantation for three days. Tiny amounts of this radioactive element are placed on the ends of metal rods, much like barbeque skewers. The rods are inserted into the vagina with the Cesium near the cancerous area in the cervix. This local approach minimizes radioactive damage to healthy tissue, unlike external radiation. The rest of each rod, about 8-inches long, remains external, lying between the patient's legs. The rods are sutured in place, and the patient must lie perfectly still. If she needs to turn, she is rolled like a log without any bending, which could cause a serious perforation. If this sounds miserable, it's because it truly is.

I entered Marne's room with admission assessment forms and was immediately blasted with words more appropriate to a locker room after a humiliating loss. It takes extreme language to impress me. In fact, just a few days before, my very own son had called me "Potty Mouth." My first thought was that the next three days would not be pleasant for Marne or the nursing staff. My second thought? How would I behave if I were under such stress and lost my inhibitions?

Marne recited her list of demands – *preferences,* I reminded myself, *preferences.* She needed organic cotton bedding and gowns. This request was easy, because we stocked those for patients with allergies. She wanted a vegan diet, also easy. The list went on. Everything needed to be natural and organic. I tried to ignore her tattoos. (Must have been organic ink.)

Back in the nursing station, I called the special orders to the linen room and dietary office, and, as I hung up, I heard a ruckus down the hall. A resident physician was in Marne's room to get permission forms signed for the surgery. From what I could hear, Marne had changed her mind about being treated. Voices escalated, and the last thing I heard from the exasperated resident as she burst out of the room was, "Well, you're going to die. Your choice!"

I went down the hall to talk with Marne; dealing with the prickly resident would have to wait. Marne had decided a radioactive implant might not fit her organic worldview. This way-out medical intervention was just too invasive for her. I excused myself and went to the break room to get a chemistry textbook. Back in Marne's room, I opened it to the Periodic Table. "Do you know what this is?" I asked.

"Yes, it's the Periodic Table."

"And what's this?" I asked, pointing to the square labeled Cs. Marne leaned in to read it.

"Cesium," she said.

"Yes," I said. "So, what could be more natural than one of the basic building blocks of nature, an element, pure and simple?"

Marne's change in attitude gave me whiplash. I couldn't believe this had worked, and I felt duplicitous. I didn't exactly trick her, and I didn't lie, but I surely did manipulate, because the periodic table does not begin to capture the experience of having metal rods inside you and poking into your thighs for three days.

I had pressured a vulnerable person. I wasn't proud of acting like that insensitive resident, but damn – Marne was going to live. Sometimes there's a real struggle between a nurse's desire to be selfless and the need to just make it through the day. Sometimes we nurses need to give ourselves the same latitude we give our patients. It helps you hang in there for the long haul, and I bet even Florence Nightingale cracked at some point. Everyone thinks that when she opened windows in stifling hospital wards, she knew fresh air was important for fighting infections. I think she just needed a good scream now and then.

When Marne returned from surgery, it took six people to keep her rigidly straight as we slid her from gurney to bed. She was not allowed to help us. A nursing student who was shadowing me stood across the bed. When we slid her sideways, Marne screamed, "What the f*** are you doing?!" A surprised nursing student heard me reply in my most calm and caring tone, "Well, Marne, what the f*** we're doing is moving you safely to the bed." If my patient spoke Spanish, I'd speak to her in Spanish. I simply spoke to Marne in Marne's native tongue. I would have enjoyed seeing the nursing student's report about "my day on the oncology unit."

Margie: Watch Your Step

One thing I enjoyed about home hospice nursing was that interlude in the car, listening to music, driving by the woods and fields, mentally finishing one visit before engaging in another. The trip to meet Margie and her brother took me well into the countryside. My directions said: *Turn on County Road 3. Watch for the rotten barn. Turn right and go 3-4 miles by the old school and wind around left at the fork. Cross the river (if the bridge has reopened) and turn into the drive by the gate. Leave your car inside the gate and walk down the path straight ahead.* The final instruction? *Walk to the gate at the far side of the field and be sure to close it or the cows will get out.* As I saw it, that put me in with the cows for much of this trek.

Maybe you're not a country person. Maybe you think cows are sweet little things like the ones that star in cottage cheese ads on TV. When you stand by an actual cow, however, especially those of the non-distaff variety, you will find they can weigh up to 2,400 lbs. I was halfway through the field when the first amorphous shapes appeared over the hill. Soon enough, those shapes became cows, and they were ambling in my direction. Eight or ten of them gathered around my shaking body. Have you ever heard cows snort? Big wet snorts with the spray backlit by the sun? I had a choice: I could keep walking or join the herd, so I shinnied along the fence to the back gate and carefully latched it as instructed.

A muddy yard surrounded the cabin. I was getting taller with each step as I gathered mud on the bottoms of my shoes. Grungy kittens appeared from under the steps and scurried around my feet, their eyes badly infected. A Cocker Spaniel came tearing around the house with teeth bared, so I placed my nursing bag between him and my knees.

When I knocked on the door, I heard a faint invitation to enter. No one was in the front room or the kitchen, so I continued to the back bedroom and found a smiling woman resting on a futon. She was pale and thin, but her face was welcoming. She appeared to be in her mid-fifties. Margie pulled back the curtain on the window over her bed and showed me the view. The cabin was close to a wide river bordered by huge weeping willows. A Great Blue Heron stood on one leg and stared at us

Margie loved being a movie producer in California, but when she became too ill to live alone, she came here to her brother's home in the Midwest. He worked the farm all day and returned to fix Margie's supper just before dark. To my surprise, she was perfectly comfortable 2,000 miles from home. I couldn't fathom the colossal jolt of moving from Rodeo Drive to the actual rodeo.

"How are you doing here alone all day?" I asked.

Margie gestured toward her books, a basket of snacks, the view outside her window. She smiled and said, "What more could you want?" This was the first of many lessons in acceptance I learned from Margie.

Over the next few months, caring for Margie was an adventure. We carried everything she needed around the cows and through the mud. This included heavy oxygen tanks, a walker, and special mattresses.

When spring brought unusually heavy rain, the river rose precipitously, breached its banks, and crept toward the cabin. We arranged for potential evacuation by boat in case of emergency or death, one of many things nursing school did not prepare me for.

"Just put me in a canoe and float me down to the Gulf of Mexico," Margie said.

I recall returning to the office after one memorable visit with Margie. It was raining hard, and as I walked back to the car, the soggy soil gripped my shoes and sucked them right off my feet. I dug them out and carried them back to the car. My pantlegs were splattered, and the rest of me didn't look so hot either. I was already late for a meeting with the hospice director, so there was no chance to clean up or change clothes. I will never forget Ellen's face when I appeared in her office doorway, dripping muddy water on her pristine carpet. There she sat, perfectly dry and well-groomed. Maybe it's good for administrators to get a glimpse of life in the trenches, though that's usually a just a metaphor. On my next visit, I shared this scene with Margie, and it made her laugh. I'm sure the producer in her was weaving this scene into a movie.

It is not easy to be torn from people and places you love, especially when you're ill and need your friends the most. I couldn't imagine what a shock Margie experienced coming to the farm, and I couldn't imagine this level of acceptance and grace. My future caregivers owe a debt of gratitude to Margie for showing me how to do it. She may have left home, but she brought everything of importance with her – her kindness, her acceptance, and her dignity.

Jenni: On Second Thought

Some terminally ill people want to remain alert and awake as long as possible, and they refuse pain medications and sedatives to the very end. Others want to be sedated from the get-go and miss the whole darn event. Some long to be left alone, while others have a party going on with friends lounging on the bed, kegs popping, and football games blaring. After witnessing the many ways life can play out from the chaotic to the sublime, I have documented my own wishes in excruciating detail. Before I engage their services, I force any new doctors to read my Durable Power of Attorney for Healthcare and assure me they will honor it. Even as I write these words, I am whispering to myself "best laid plans."

ALS (amyotrophic lateral sclerosis) slowly disables motor muscle movements, often leaving the mind intact, but the body frozen, unable to make even the slightest move. It is especially important for someone facing this debility to make his nor her wishes clear to family and healthcare professionals before communication is compromised. Jenni, who in her early forties was young for an ALS patient, clearly understood the importance of making her wishes known. Before she signed admission forms to hospice, she wanted to know that we understood and would respect her decisions. I put down my clipboard and listened. Jenni said she had a plan to end her life when she could no longer speak or write by hand, and she had a few buddies who'd agreed to help her. A successful lyricist and composer, Jenni said that, for her, the stroke of a pencil was an integral part of creating music, and she was not the least bit interested in exploring assistive devices. I took a moment to compose my thoughts, then told her this would not prevent me from admitting her.

This young woman just told me she planned to commit suicide when she no longer could hold a pencil, so why didn't I press the issue? Because in my experience, people usually *approach* the point they think will be unbearable or devoid of meaning, but seldom do they *reach* it. Life keeps reinventing value and meaning for them. The line in the sand keeps blowing down the beach. It's not that I didn't believe Jenni was committed to her plan, but it's not worth getting your stethoscope in a knot when stepping into such a complex, ever-changing situation.

As I left Jenni's house, I thought about where I'd draw my own line. I already had a mental list of things to keep me warm and comfortable when I decide it's time to slip quietly into Lake Michigan for my last kayak ride. It'll happen before dawn, and I'll have music and a thermos of tea, maybe my mother's old hot water bottle and a quilt. Probably some good drugs, too. Yet deep down, I know that I, like almost everyone else, won't quite know when it's time to push off.

Jenni was confined to a wheelchair and needed help with basic cares, but she spent her days writing with enthusiasm and enjoyment. As the months went on, she shared some of the songs she was working on. Her lyrics were beautiful poems, and her melodies haunting and poignant.

Sadly, ALS cannot be deterred, and day by day, it claimed more of her mobility. This was a delicate time, because the pencil had indeed fallen from Jenni's hand for the last time. Despite the best efforts of her devoted friends, staying home became impossible. Round-the-clock "care by committee" seldom is sustainable over the long haul. Would she put her end-of-life plan into action?

With no mention of the plan, Jenni decided to move to a care center. Over time, she took on a new mission: lying in a nursing home bed, communicating with nothing except blinks, she dedicated herself to teaching caregivers how to work with someone in her situation. She taught them to take their time and to talk to her, not to her disability. All this she managed by opening and closing her eyes, a painfully slow way to communicate. This successful composer and lyricist told me her new role as teacher was the most rewarding of her life, that her legacy was educating this crew of physicians, nurses, and aides.

The entire staff appreciated Jenni's strength and openness of heart. It turns out that in the blink of an eye, she had bestowed gifts that would benefit countless others. Jenni's legacy, like her music, will keep on singing.

Daniel: The Finale

Marta was unresponsive, lying motionless in a hospital bed in the living room of her small Cape Cod house. Her skin was remarkably smooth for a woman in her 80s, and her silky white hair shimmered in the sunlight streaming through the picture window. Marta was the picture of a peaceful, comfortable woman taking a nap, but her breathing and blood pressure indicated she was very close to death.

The home was simple, decorated with family pictures and keepsakes from trips. The piano across the room was stacked with sheet music, and in the corner stood a music stand and violin case. Such a beautiful, homey setting to wrap-up a long life.

Marta's husband, Daniel, had been a music teacher. His face sagged with sadness, and he was both tired and squeezed dry by grief. I assured him he was doing a wonderful job caring for his wife. He wondered if there was a reason she was holding on so long, worried that she was suffering. I asked if she might be waiting for someone or if something might be unresolved. Daniel could think of nothing. Their adult children had said their goodbyes, and good friends had visited faithfully these last few days.

Daniel was a gentle, thoughtful man, and when he talked about their long life together, tears filled his eyes. I asked if Marta had a favorite song he might play for her. His face brightened, pleased there was something more he could do. He sat at the piano and played softly, tenderly, and I watched his posture straighten a bit.

As Daniel played and hummed the hymn, "In the Garden," I

noticed Marta's face slacken. When he finished the hymn, I touched his shoulder, and he turned to me.

"She's gone?" he asked. I nodded. He went to his wife and took her hands, laying his cheek against hers. Years before, in a pet store, I'd seen a lovebird clinging to its perch, leaning at an odd angle. The store owner told me that after the bird's partner died, the bird continued to lean in as though his mate were still next to him. I knew Daniel would lean toward Marta for the rest of his life.

"What now?" he asked. He wasn't ready to be done, not after sixty-five years together.

"Would you like to wash her face, Daniel?" I asked.

"Oh, yes!" he said, relieved the end was still a few minutes off. I brought him a basin of warm water. Daniel took the washcloth and stroked Marta's face, and I waited around the corner as he spent this last moment with his wife. He told her he loved her, and she was a good mother and wife. He washed her hands and patted them dry, then nodded to me, his goodbye complete. Who wouldn't like to finish his or her life like this – loved, clean, and dignified, listening to a favorite song played by someone you love?

Hospice nurses walk into many chaotic, dramatic situations, but this was a sweet, quiet scene. Here was this unremarkable, unassuming man in his average house doing the hardest thing of all: being there, no matter how difficult. Some acts of bravery are so simple we may not notice them. Many heroes fly well under the radar.

Being allowed into such moments in the life of a stranger is something you cannot explain to those who think your work is boring or gross or demeaning. I admit to being an intensity junkie, attracted to difficult situations, relishing the challenge of bringing calm to a storm, but a quiet and beautiful conclusion to a life like Marta's is a pretty good fix, too.

Edna: Cold Comfort

Ice storms are no deterrent to an on-call hospice nurse, but the drive to Edna's home did include a few fishtails and one slide through a stop sign. The telltale porch light on an otherwise dark street identified the house where I was expected in the middle of the night. The elderly woman had died before the family called, so I was here to comfort, tie up loose ends, and deal with the funeral home.

A long, icy sidewalk sloped up to the front door. I should have worn cleats. Instead, I skated along on smooth-soled tennies and grabbed onto shrubs to pull myself up to the porch. My feet shot sideways and around in circles.

When I reached the door, I clawed through my wind-blown hair before I rang the bell. A middle-aged gentleman opened the door and invited me in. His wife and two small children watched from the living room.

"I'm sorry about your mom," I said.

"Nothin' we didn't expect," he answered, his tone ending the conversation like the slice of a knife. "Grandma's upstairs." He nodded toward the stairway in the corner. This wasn't any old stairway. It was a self-contained, iron column – tall and narrow with triangular steps winding around a central pole. I was delivered into the upstairs through a hole in the ceiling.

Grandma, a short, full-figured woman, lay in a low twin bed, so it wasn't going to be easy lifting her. I carried out my duties and then called the funeral home. They said they'd be on their way, and I wound my way back downstairs to the living room where the family sat silently. There are many different responses to death, so a nurse must proceed with caution. When my attempts at conversation fell flat, I let things be, because there was no way to know if this was their usual style, if there was an abuse history, or any number of possibilities. I was relieved when the doorbell rang and ran to greet the man from the funeral home. It was not the usual guy.

"Omigod, the ice," he said. He was a skinny needle of a man, red faced and shivering with the cold. Clearly, he wasn't used to these middle-of-the-night runs to pick up bodies. I poked my head out the door and looked around, because funeral homes always send two guys.

"Came alone," he said. "Busy night." My back throbbed at the thought of the two of us carrying Grandma.

"Where's the gurney?" I asked.

"Right here," he said, pointing at some long, wooden poles he was holding. Turns out, he'd brought a WWI era stretcher consisting of two poles with a piece of canvas in between.

"All the regular gurneys are in use," he said. He handed me the poles and took off his black topcoat. Clearly, the situation was not going to improve, because he had only one arm.

I pointed at the staircase and led the way. Once upstairs, I looked down at this man as he struggled with the stretcher, banging the poles on every rung, hitting himself on the forehead, and somehow getting everything jammed sideways. I went down a few steps, dislodged him, and led the way down the hall to the bedroom.

"Oh, my," he said when he saw the grandmother, who was twice his size. We rolled her to the side of the bed, and I held her there while he unfurled his canvas and laid it on the sheet. I rolled Grandma back. Didn't know what kind of wood those poles were made of, but I surely hoped they would support this woman all the way to the funeral home station wagon without incident. We covered her with a sheet and fastened two wide straps to hold her to the stretcher.

"One, two three," I said. We lifted, inched our way out of the room, and crept forward, my helper turning beet red from the effort. Down the hall, the menacing hole in the floor awaited us. I hoisted my end of the stretcher onto my right shoulder, grabbed the handrail, and took one step down, which put us at about ten degrees off horizontal. I moved down another step. Twenty degrees off horizontal. Third step – and so it went. Now, back behind me, or more accurately up above me, it was funeral man's turn to take his first step down. He hoisted the stretcher onto his shoulder and held it there, leaning his hip against the rail for support. I proceeded downward, my knees shaking, buckling under the full weight of the stretcher (and for all I knew, the funeral man.) Of course, there was no reason those poles would go down any easier than they had come up. We got snagged on every wrought-iron grape leaf and hummingbird. Halfway down, our load was nearly vertical. Old movie scenes flashed through my mind, the ones where a sailor dies mid-journey, where they put him on a plank, tip it over the rail, and slide the body into the ocean. This alarming image helped me stay strong, because Edna's grandchildren were watching the scene unfold.

We made it downstairs without traumatizing anyone, and Edna's son opened the front door for us. I led the way. We stepped onto the front porch and immediately began sliding down the sidewalk toward the black station wagon, picking up speed as we went, racing toward the car while the family watched from the doorway. When I smacked into the side of the car, the funeral home man fell flat on his back behind me. The stretcher landed on top of him and then sliced into my Achilles tendons, flinging me backward onto the pile. We three rested halfway under the car, half out in the elements, looking up at falling snow.

I heard the front door shut, and the porch light went out. When Grandma was tucked safely inside the station wagon, funeral man

smiled and waved as he drove off. I sat in my car while it warmed up and called in report to our recorded line.
 "Mrs. Goodman died. Otherwise, a quiet night."

David: Facing the Music

Head and neck cancers are among the most difficult for everyone concerned – patients, families, and those who treat and care for them. They threaten vital functions such as breathing and eating. They can compromise hearing, vision, the sense of smell and the ability to taste. Disease and treatments can affect speech and appearance, impacting relationships and social activities.

David reluctantly allowed his exhausted, stressed-out wife to call hospice, and she met us in the living room of their modest ranch home. On the end table, there was a framed photo of David, his wife, and their adult son. David, now 60, was about 40 in the photo, a tall man with wavy hair and high cheek bones. His eyes were Paul Newman blue with a flirtatious little squint.

David's wife invited us to sit for a moment before we met him. Talking *about* instead of *with* a patient made me uneasy. Imagine lying in bed, hearing people talking about you in the next room. It's as though you are not an adult with feelings or a say in your own life. The wife informed us David agreed to this meeting with hospice only at her insistence. He was refusing to see friends, allowed only a dim light in his room, and spent all his time in bed. In addition to threatening his life, parotid gland cancer radically changed David's appearance, and he wouldn't allow his son to visit, fearing it would disturb him.

After twenty-minutes, David agreed to meet me, probably wanting to know what we were saying about him. I found a thin man, turned toward the wall. His scalp was caved in as was one eyebrow ridge. A large scar ran in front of David's ear, the location of the parotid gland, and his skin was darkened by radiation treatments. It wasn't easy for him to speak, because with a major salivary gland destroyed and radiation damage, dry mouth was severe.

David required extensive care, and his wife was doing a good job. She cleansed and packed wounds and dealt with suctioning secretions to prevent choking and skin erosion. Emotional support, however, was non-existent for either of them.

The hospice team of physicians, nurses, social workers, chaplain, and aides went to work. After a month, David's emotional state hadn't improved, so another team member was summoned. Because I'd seen a guitar in the corner of his room, I asked David to try one session with our music therapist and promised that if he didn't enjoy it, I wouldn't mention it again. He said she could come if she didn't enter the bedroom.

Peggy sang and played guitar in the living room, and after a few sessions, David did invite her into his room. A baritone in his barbershop quartet, he couldn't resist singing along, and within a few weeks, David was sitting on his couch, singing duets with Peggy. Together, they wrote a beautiful song for his wife, which Peggy sang at David's funeral.

Music therapy profoundly impacted this family, and I call that a major medical miracle. Sometimes medicine and nursing need to get out of the way and watch the real healing take place.

Annie: A Father's Gift

Being on-call means being pulled away from Thanksgiving dinner, crawling out of a warm bed to negotiate a blizzard or missing a spouse's birthday or a nephew's wedding. Still, there are many things I appreciated about being on-call for hospice. Coming into a chaotic situation and bringing some relief is very satisfying. I also loved having the full force of the *hospice way* behind me, meaning if someone required emotional care or support related to family dynamics, they deserved a visit as much as someone having a physical crisis, even at 3:00 a.m. This is rewarding for a nurse, being able to provide the care her patient deserves without battling the system.

One of the more difficult on-call situations is visiting a family you have not met, especially if there is a crisis or a death. This was the case when I was called to Annie's home.

She was a young mom of three little girls. I heard about Annie in our weekly team meetings. She was one of those people always trying to make things easier for other people, a fun-loving person, someone who threw epic backyard parties. She sang in a women's chorus and was teaching her girls to sing, creating her own little trio. When struck down by cancer, she was the one comforting friends and family. She spent every minute she could with her girls.

I was greeted by Annie's husband, Carlos, a man in such pain his voice was barely audible. He showed me to her hospital bed in the living room. Annie was near death, her breathing slow and shallow. She appeared to be comfortable, but her husband was not. He was in anguish. He paced and fussed with things on the bedside table, and I could tell he needed to do something, anything. After a few minutes, he said he wanted to take her to the hospital. With a little encouragement, he explained that he was afraid the girls would see their mom die in a home where they would grow up without her.

I knew the transfer to a stretcher and ride to the hospital might cause Annie pain, and if she awakened, confusion and fear. It would be terrible if she died en route. Furthermore, I knew that in the ER, she might be stowed behind a curtain, because they rightly prioritize saving lives. I tried to communicate this without adding to Carlos' distress and to affirm he could take his wife to the hospital if that's what he chose to do. He listened, and without explanation, went outside and stood on the patio, peering into the darkness.

When Carlos returned, he did something unexpected: he awakened the girls, who were ten, seven, and six, brought them to the living room, and asked them to sing to their mom. Half asleep, they did their best to sing, "You've Got a Friend in Me." Tears streamed down the oldest child's face. When they finished, Carlos said, "You were very brave, and I know you made your mom happy." He took them back down the hall and tucked them into bed.

Annie died an hour later, a loss beyond measure for this family. Carlos had sacrificed his own comfort for his girls. I knew they'd be fine in his care, and I'm sure Annie knew, too.

Ida: Hide the Kids!

Some patients remain in my heart because they mustered exceptional grace in their last days, weathering pain, fear, and indignity with bravery. On the other hand, there's a special corner of my heart reserved for the feistier folks, the ones who do not "go gentle into that good night." They go out and tear up yard signs and shoot out streetlights. They beat the gentle right outta that good night. Ida was one of those feisty ones.

Ida was in her last summer. She was mad at her cancer and the world in general. In her seventies, she lived alone with adult children nearby. She was thin. I could have put a finger under her chin and lifted her off the ground, but she still managed to care for her house and run short errands. Ida, however, grew weaker every day, and her dose of pain meds was rising, so it wouldn't be long before she needed help.

Someone in Ida's condition should never think of getting behind the wheel, so when she backed her massive Buick down the driveway, you wanted to yell, "Get all the kids in the house!" One day, Ida's daughter asked the hospice team to make her mom stop driving. People are never tickled when you ask them to stop driving, and it's even less popular when you're an outsider. We suggested some things her family might try before we got involved.

First attempt: Ida's children expressed their concern and asked her to call whenever she needed a ride. They said they'd be happy to come. She smiled and nodded and had no intention of accepting their offer. Second attempt, they drew straws. Youngest son, Ted, got the short one and took her keys away. Ida ran him off the porch, screaming something about his inheritance. Then she had a new set of keys made. (This is when I fell in love with Ida, largely because I know this is how I will face my own demise.)

A few weeks passed, and Ida was now receiving a significant dose of morphine. Her mobility was limited – she barely could raise a foot to hit the brake pedal. In desperation, Ida's son removed the spark plugs from her car. He told her it wouldn't run, that it was unrepairable. She took it well, and after lunch, she had the Buick towed in and the spark plugs replaced. The ornery cheerleader inside me did cartwheels for Ida. On the other hand, her house was not far from the hospice office, so I planned to stay off the street when she was out and about.

Though they'd rather have poked an irritable tiger, Ida's family decided to sell her car. I felt sad for her. Giving up driving means a loss of freedom and independence. Of course, it was the right thing to do, since she was a danger to herself and anyone on the sidewalk. The deed was done. The Buick was sold.

This was not one of those feel-good moments in nursing. Ida felt ganged up on by her family and the hospice team. To her credit, she did not wallow in self-pity; she simply went out and bought a new car.

When my adult children come shuffling up the driveway looking guilty, I'll think about you, Ida – your determination and your spunk. Meanwhile, I'm hiding my spare set of keys.

Margaret: The Special Gift

Some patients connect with you in a way that changes you as a nurse and as a person. Margaret was such a woman. She came to the oncology unit wearing sensible shoes and a stern expression, her mahogany hair in a short, no-nonsense hairstyle. Margaret's eyes were bright green with long, dark lashes. This was a beautiful, middle-aged woman, albeit one who was strictly business. A penetrating intelligence emanated from her face. (I had recently graduated from nursing school at 41, the same age as Margaret. She was my first primary patient, meaning I was responsible for planning and coordinating her care and for providing it when I was on duty.)

Margaret had advanced ovarian cancer, but she did not let this frightening diagnosis and poor prognosis deter her from her work. Fully cognizant of the serious nature of her cancer, she thought this disease was a nuisance, something interrupting her busy schedule. This was not someone accustomed to being out of control. She refused a hospital gown, remained dressed for business, and worked while we administered chemotherapy.

Margaret was curt and deep voiced, and she often caused me to fumble the few answers I knew as a recent grad. One of our first encounters went especially badly. I gave Margaret an intramuscular injection, a shot deep into the muscle with a long needle. We tried to use less painful routes of delivery for medications, but unfortunately, this drug could not be given in an IV. Margaret rolled over and waited. I thought the injection went well. She, however, rose out of bed like Shamu and snarled at me, "That was the worst injection ever!" It takes some determination to re-enter a patient's room after such an incident. I figured I had blown what little trust I'd established.

Over the next few months, Margaret spiraled downward, a predictable pattern for her type and stage of cancer. Her disease was Lord and Master, and though the medical staff threw their best armaments at it, her tumor raged back. We knew it would win, as did Margaret, but she kept working at the table in her hospital room. Her attitude was, "Do what you have to do and let me get on with business." This became more and more difficult, because over time, Margaret did not tolerate her treatments well. Inevitable complications created undignified situations for this very dignified woman, and hospital stays became more frequent.

Over the summer, Margaret and I developed a close relationship, and as I learned more, I earned her trust. I was fascinated by her strength, and she was puzzled by my desire to work in this "horrifying world," as she described it. We talked during her infusions, sometimes in the middle of the night. She remained tough if you screwed up, and she often made me feel I had. I found her interesting, complex, and in her own way, kind.

As Margaret entered the last phase of her illness, she experimented on her own with new approaches to this nightmare thrust upon her. At home, she hired a spiritual guide, she learned meditation, and had regular massages, acupressure, and therapeutic touch. These were "out there" therapies for such a logic-driven woman. On her last visit, she was aware of her impending death, and I saw a sweeter, more mellow Margaret.

One night at 2:30 a.m., Margaret's call light came on. She reported severe back pain, so I increased her morphine dose, but I could see her emotional pain was as severe as her physical pain. Clearly, she was afraid. I admired this woman, loved her. I told her I'd check with the other nurse, and if I could, would return to give her a back massage. Two of us were caring for fourteen critically ill patients, but luckily, it was an unusually quiet night. My colleague would come find me if things started revving up.

I'd recently completed a course in therapeutic touch at Brigham and Women's Hospital in Boston. Since then, my only opportunity to practice was on our puzzled Australian Shepherd. I stood outside Margaret's door, debating, while images of pressure points on laminated charts danced in my head. I was a novice, and I was sure Margaret would let me know how far from therapeutic my touch was. I decided not to mention my Boston internship or what I was attempting to do. To be safe, I'd call it a plain old massage.

The room was quiet except for the hum of the IV pump. I sat at the head of the bed and massaged Margaret's shoulders, upper arms, and the back of her head. I felt for pressure points, pressing and releasing, massaging into them. I could feel Margaret softening.

By the end of our session, Margaret was still, her respirations slow. She was in a deeply relaxed state. And there it was – that intersection, that strong connection between patient and nurse, obviating the question, "How can you stand to be a nurse?" I could stand it because this dear woman was in a relaxed and peaceful place.

I tiptoed to the door, and as I stepped into the hallway, Margaret gave me a profoundly generous gift. She spoke from within her trance, whispering, "Thank you for learning to do that." Not "thank you for *doing* that" but "thank you for *learning* to do that." Precise to the end, Margaret used her precious energy to go beyond thanking me: she perceived and acknowledged the effort I'd taken to prepare myself. Yes, Margaret, I can, indeed, stand to be a nurse. In fact, I am most grateful to be a nurse.

Acknowledgements

I wish to acknowledge and honor my nurse colleagues. Even while scraping things off their shoes or enduring deadly in-services, they were determined to be excellent nurses and strong advocates. My hospital and hospice colleagues remain treasured friends years later. If you are a nursing student, be assured that you are heading somewhere special. Your long hours, effort, and frustration will be worth the trip, more than you can imagine.

I also thank my excellent writing teachers from high school to this very day for bolstering my skills and my confidence. My uniquely congenial writing group holds my toes to the line with skill, love, and understanding. (Thank you, Mary, Amy, Bettye Jo, and Wendy, Jr.) Thank you also to friends and relatives who have endured endless first drafts and helped me get some to the finish line. Some say writing is a lonely task, but not for me.

I am indebted to those patients and families who let me into their lives at such challenging times. You, too, were my teachers, and you remain embedded in my heart.

For this opportunity and for wisdom and guidance, I am grateful to:

- Michigan Writers Cooperative Press and managing Editor, Bruce Makie
- Contest readers
- Editor, Julie Bonner Williams
- Judge, Phillip Sterling
- Artist/Designer, Amy Hansen

About the Creative Nonfiction Judge

Phillip Sterling is an essayist, poet and fiction writer. He is the recipient of a National Endowment for the Arts Fellowship in Poetry, two Senior Fulbright Lectureships, A PEN Syndicated Fiction Award, and artist in residences at Isle Royale National Park and Sleeping Bear Dunes. Raised in Traverse City, Phillip is professor emeritus at Ferris State University. His latest work, *Lessons in Geography/The Education of a Michigan Poet,* is a warm, sprawling and humorous memoir.

About the Author

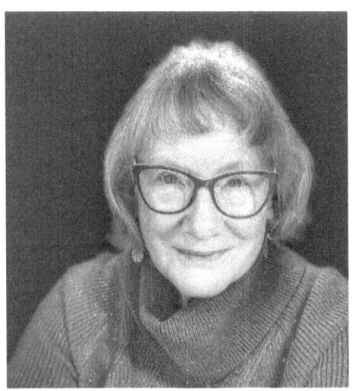

Wendy Gilbert Gronbeck lives and writes on the dunes above Lake Michigan. She writes memoir, short stories, flash, and essays. Ms. Gronbeck has worked as a video producer and writer, an oncology nurse and hospice nurse. These varied careers have provided first-hand experience with trauma and grief, heroism, and humor; her themes and characters are born of that experience. Ms. Gronbeck's work has appeared in Our Iowa Magazine; Michigan History Magazine; her blogs–*Iowa County Almanac, Living in the Country, and Woody and the Widow;* the Erma Bombeck and Little Old Lady Comedy blogs; the short story anthology, *Revenge* (Free Spirit, 2022.) Her novel, *Drownings,* was a finalist in Novel Slices 2022, The Institute for the Novel. Her flash stories, *Shooting and Still,* appeared in The Bangalore Press and The New Plains Review, respectively. For more about Wendy, please go to wendygilbertgronbeck.com

About Michigan Writers Cooperative Press

This book was published in the spring of 2025 in a signed edition of 100 copies.

This chapbook is part of the Cooperative Series of the Michigan Writers Small Press Project, which was launched in 2005 to give members of Michigan Writers, Inc. a new avenue to publication. All of the chapbooks in this series are an author's first book in that genre. The Cooperative Press shoulders the publishing costs for the first edition, and writers share the marketing and promotional responsibilities in return for the prestige of being published by a press that prints only carefully selected manuscripts.

Chapbook length manuscripts of poetry, short stories, and essays are solicited each year from members and adjudicated by a panel of experienced writers and a judge who is a specialist in a particular genre. For more information, please visit www.michwriters.org.

MICHIGAN WRITERS is an open-membership organization dedicated to providing opportunities for networking, professional growth, and publication for writers of all ages and skill levels in the state of Michigan and beyond.

EDITOR: Julie Bonner Williams

MANAGING EDITOR: Bruce L. Makie

BOOK DESIGN: Amy Hansen

Other Titles Available
from Michigan Writers Cooperative Press

The Grace of the Eye by Michael Callaghan
Trouble With Faces by Trinna Frever
Box of Echoes by Todd Mercer
Beyond the Reach of Imagination by Duncan Spratt Moran
The Grass Impossibly by Holly Wren Spaulding
The Chocolatier Speaks of his Wife by Catherine Turnbull
Dangerous Exuberance by Leigh Fairey
Point of Sand by Jaimien Delp
Hard Winter, First Thaw by Jenny Robertson
Friday Nights the Whole Town Goes to the Basketball Game by Teresa J. Scollon
Seasons for Growing by Sarah Baughman
Forking the Swift by Jennifer Sperry Steinorth
The Rest of Us by John Mauk
Kisses for Laura by Joan Schmeichel
Eat the Apple by Denise Baker
First Risings by Michael Hughes
Fathers and Sons by Bruce L. Makie
Exit Wounds by Jim Crockett
The Solid Living World by Ellen Stone
Bitter Dagaa by Robb Astor
Crime Story by Kris Kuntz
Michaela by Gabriella Burman
Supposing She Dreamed This by Gail Wallace Bozzano
Line and Hook by Kevin Griffin
And Sarah His Wife by Christina Diane Campbell
Proud Flesh by Nancy Parshall
Angel Rides a Bike by Margaret Fedder
Ink by Kathleen Pfeiffer
What Will You Teach Her? by Megan Klco Kellner
Bluetongue and Other Michigan Stories by Ryan Shek
The Mountain Ash by Kathleen Rabbers
This Blue Earth by Sharon Bippus
Upstairs, Listening by Melinda LePere
Twinkies by Kathleen Quigley
The Sound a Car Door Makes by Natalie Tomlin
Brain Aura Blues by Melissa Seitz
Bones and Breath by Ruth Zwald

**Michigan
WRITERS**

www.ingramcontent.com/pod-product-compliance
Lightning Source LLC
Chambersburg PA
CBHW060543080526
44586CB00012B/837